ANA PATRICIA DE OLIVEIRA
JANAINA MAIA LIMA ROSAL
BRUNA DA SILVA SOUZA

LIVER SYSTEM:

ANA PATRICIA DE OLIVEIRA
JANAINA MAIA LIMA ROSAL
BRUNA DA SILVA SOUZA

LIVER SYSTEM:

Its importance and treatment

ScienciaScripts

Imprint

Any brand names and product names mentioned in this book are subject to trademark, brand or patent protection and are trademarks or registered trademarks of their respective holders. The use of brand names, product names, common names, trade names, product descriptions etc. even without a particular marking in this work is in no way to be construed to mean that such names may be regarded as unrestricted in respect of trademark and brand protection legislation and could thus be used by anyone.

Cover image: www.ingimage.com

This book is a translation from the original published under ISBN 978-620-6-76040-5.

Publisher:
Sciencia Scripts
is a trademark of
Dodo Books Indian Ocean Ltd. and OmniScriptum S.R.L publishing group

120 High Road, East Finchley, London, N2 9ED, United Kingdom
Str. Armeneasca 28/1, office 1, Chisinau MD-2012, Republic of Moldova, Europe
Printed at: see last page
ISBN: 978-620-7-66544-0

CHAPTER 1

LIVER SYSTEM

ANA PATRICIA DE OLIVEIRA JANAINA MAIA LIMA ROSAL
BRUNA DA SILVA SOUZA
ALESSANDRA MARIA BRAGA RIBEIRO NAYLSON DE JESUS
RIBEIRO
MARIA EDUARDA FERNANDES ARAUJO

The liver is the second largest organ, second only to the skin, and the largest gland in the human body. It performs several essential functions for the body to function, such as eliminating toxic substances and producing bile, an essential product for digesting fats. One of the diseases that affect the liver is cirrhosis, which can be caused by alcoholism and diseases such as hepatitis B and C.

Liver functions

The liver is an organ with important functions. This organ is considered to be a connecting region between the digestive system and the blood, where nutrients absorbed in the digestive tract are processed and stored for later distribution to other organs. Nutrients from the intestine reach the liver via the portal vein, with the exception of complex lipids, which arrive via the hepatic artery. With regard to carbohydrates, the liver is responsible for storing large quantities of glycogen. This storage is important for controlling glucose levels in the blood, since storage in the form of glycogen ensures that glucose is withdrawn when it is in excess, and in situations where there is a drop in glucose levels, the stored glycogen is degraded and released, ensuring an increase in glucose levels in the blood.

It's worth noting that blood coming from the intestine is often full of bacteria. The liver works to kill these bacteria as the blood passes through by the sinusoids. The so-called Kupffer cells are macrophages capable of phagocytising foreign organisms that arrive at the site, and are therefore fundamental in controlling bacteria.

It is in the liver that bile is synthesised, usually between 600 mL/day and 1000 mL/day. Bile is a substance made up of salts, which act as emulsifiers, causing large particles of fat to be reduced to smaller particles, which will be attacked by the lipases present in the pancreatic juice.

For this reason, even though it doesn't contain enzymes, bile plays an important role in the digestion of fats. In addition, the salts present in it help absorb the products of fat digestion through the intestinal mucosa. After being synthesised in the liver, bile is stored in the gallbladder. During the production of bile, the liver incorporates by-products of the destruction of red blood cells (the liver ensures the destruction of old red blood cells), such as bilirubin. This pigment is then eliminated from the body via faeces. When there is too much bilirubin in the blood, the skin and mucous membranes turn yellow, a condition known as jaundice. The liver also ensures the production of plasma proteins such as albumin and fibrinogen. It also stores vitamins, most notably vitamin A. It also stores iron in the form of ferritin. The liver is also responsible for removing or excreting medicines, hormones and other substances. In the embryo, the liver is responsible for producing red blood cells. The liver performs important functions in various processes in the body. These include: filtering micro-organisms: the organ is one of the main responsible for the body's immune defence; detoxifying the body: the liver transforms hormones and drugs into non-active substances so that they can be excreted by the body, preventing poisoning; transforming ammonia into urea: if the organ is damaged, ammonia will pass into the circulation and reach the brain, causing neuropsychic changes (behavioural changes, forgetfulness, insomnia, drowsiness) and coma, secrete bile: bile is a fluid that acts in the digestion of fats and the absorption o f nutritious substances; store glucose: glucose is the main source of energy for the body. the functioning of other organs; producing proteins: the liver is responsible for producing proteins linked to the blood clotting process, and also for producing albumin, which helps transport substances through the bloodstream.

CHAPTER 2

MAIN LIVER DISEASES AND INJURIES

ANA PATRICIA DE OLIVEIRA JANAINA MAIA LIMA ROSAL
BRUNA DA SILVA SOUZA

Most liver problems have similar symptoms because, even though they have different origins, these diseases compromise the same functions of the organ.

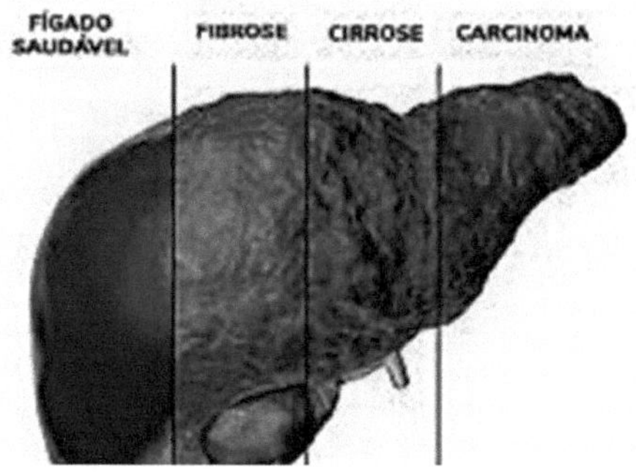

Source:

The symptoms listed here may have other origins, and do not necessarily indicate liver disease. However, it is important to see a doctor if any of these symptoms appear:

o Jaundice: a yellowish tinge to the eyes and skin.

o Ascites: accumulation   within the abdominal cavity, known as popularly known as water belly.

o Digestive bleeding and sudden haemorrhagic vomiting.

o Encephalopathy: alteration of basic brain functions, which can cause lethargy, irritability, difficulty concentrating, reduced level of consciousness and coma.

o Gynaecomastia: development of breasts in men

o Telangiectasias: vascular lesions known as vascular spiders. They are most often found on the trunk, face and arms.

o Pain or swelling in the upper right part of the abdomen, below the ribs.

But long before these symptoms appear, your body can show signs that suggest liver problems are beginning:

o Itchy body

o Tiredness or discouragement

o Motion sickness after meals

o Dizziness, headache, fever, excessive sweating, difficulty concentrating

o Redness in the palm of the hand and the appearance of purple spots on the skin

o Clearer faeces

o Nosebleeds

o Abnormal bleeding after minor trauma

o Dry mouth, bitter taste in the mouth

o Constipation or diarrhoea

o Excessive weight gain or loss for no reason

These signs are non-specific and can simply be the result of changes in your routine or eating habits. Always see your doctor if you experience a large number of symptoms at the same time, if some of them occur frequently or if they persist for a long time.

Types of liver disease

There are several liver diseases and, as we've already said, the symptoms can be very similar. The difference between them is usually the severity and speed with which they damage the liver. A lack of research can lead many doctors to diagnose more traditional diseases such as viral hepatitis too early. This error is unacceptable. The suspicion of a liver disease should be investigated comprehensively with imaging tests, biopsies and laboratory tests.

The main diseases affecting the liver include:

Hepatic steatosis

Hepatic steatosis is a disorder characterised by the accumulation of fat inside hepatocytes (liver cells) - an organ located on the right side of the abdomen through which a large amount of blood circulates. Reddish-brown in colour, the liver performs more than 500 fundamental functions for the body.The constant and prolonged increase in fat within the hepatocytes can cause inflammation that can develop into serious cases of fatty hepatitis, liver cirrhosis and even cancer. In these cases, the liver not only increases in size, but also takes on a yellowish appearance.

Also known as fatty liver disease, fatty liver or fatty liver, hepatic steatosis is an increasingly common condition, which can also manifest itself in childhood and affects more women. It is estimated that 30 per cent of the population has the problem and that approximately half of all sufferers can progress to more serious forms of the disease.

Hepatic steatosis can be categorised as alcoholic (caused by excessive alcohol consumption) and non-alcoholic. Overweight, diabetes, poor nutrition, sudden weight loss, pregnancy, surgery and a sedentary lifestyle are all risk factors for the appearance of non-alcoholic fatty liver steatosis. There is evidence that metabolic syndrome (high blood pressure, insulin resistance, high cholesterol and triglyceride levels) and abdominal obesity are directly associated with excess fat cells in the liver.

In a much smaller number of cases, thin, abstemious people with no changes in cholesterol or glycaemia can develop fatty liver steatosis.

In children in the first few years of life, hepatic steatosis is mainly caused by some metabolic diseases (causing alterations in the functioning of the liver). the body in general). In older children and adolescents, the causes are similar to those of adults. Treatment in childhood is of fundamental importance to prevent irreversible damage in adults, as well as raising children's awareness of healthy lifestyle habits.

Symptoms:

In mild cases of hepatic steatosis, the disease doesn't cause any symptoms; these are only noticed when the complications of the disease appear. Initially, the complaints are pain, tiredness, weakness, loss of appetite and enlargement of the liver. In the more advanced stages of steatohepatitis, characterised by inflammation and fibrosis resulting in liver failure, the most frequent symptoms are ascites (abnormal accumulation of fluid inside the abdomen), encephalopathy (diseases of the brain) and mental confusion, haemorrhages, a drop in the number of platelets in the blood, jaundice (yellowing of the skin and eyes).

Diagnosis:

In the early stages, the diagnosis of non-alcoholic fatty steatohepatitis is often made by means of routine laboratory or imaging tests. Once the alteration has been detected, it is essential to establish a differential diagnosis with other hepatitis, autoimmune and genetic diseases, or drug use, since the disease does not have a characteristic clinical picture. If suspicion arises, however, the important thing is to take the patient's history, carry out a thorough physical examination and undergo blood tests to measure liver enzyme levels. Although ultrasound, tomography and magnetic resonance imaging are very useful for assessing possible alterations in the liver, there are cases in which confirmation of the diagnosis depends on a biopsy. However, the most important test for diagnosing the disease is transient elastography, a painless method similar to ultrasound that measures the elasticity of liver tissue and the amount of fat accumulated in the liver.

Treatment:

There is no specific treatment for excess fatty liver. It is determined according to the causes of the disease, which is curable, and is based on three pillars: a healthy lifestyle, a balanced diet and regular exercise. Rarely is it necessary to introduce medication.

Prevention:

Some measures are essential to prevent the accumulation of fat in the liver or to reverse the condition that has already set in. Some parameters are used as a possible risk group, such as: abdominal circumference measurements, which should not exceed 88 cm in women, and 102 cm in men; keep your weight within the ideal standards for your height and age, but be careful, radical diets that cause you to lose weight too quickly can make the condition worse; drink in moderation (alcoholic drinks) during the week and at weekends too; reduce your consumption of refined carbohydrates and saturated fats. Replace them with wholemeal foods and olive oil, fish, fruit and vegetables.

Cirrhosis

Liver cirrhosis is a condition in which the normal histological architecture of the liver is altered, with an increase in connective tissue and the formation of scar tissue. It is considered the main chronic disease affecting the organ. Its causes are varied, such as excessive alcohol consumption, autoimmune liver diseases and viral hepatitis (B and C).Cirrhosis can cause different symptoms, such as swelling in the legs, weight loss, loss of appetite, weakness, fluid accumulation in the abdomen (ascites), yellowing of the skin and mucous membranes (jaundice), cramps, tremors and mental confusion. The diagnosis is made by analysing the patient's symptoms and by laboratory and imaging tests, such as ultrasound and CT scans. A liver biopsy should also be carried out.It's worth pointing out that, so far, the only way to cure the problem is through liver transplantation. Medications can help slow down the progression, but they do not lead to a cure. It is important that changes in the liver are treated early to prevent cirrhosis from developing.Also called cirrhosis of the liver, cirrhosis is a condition in which some liver cells are destroyed or stop functioning properly, resulting in the formation of scars, fibrosis and nodules in the tissue and causing the liver to function impaired or partially affected.Cirrhosis is the consequence of a series of inflammatory processes that have affected the liver in the past. As the organ goes through these processes, changes occur in its tissue. Once this tissue becomes so altered that the organ is unable to function properly, the patient is diagnosed with cirrhosis. The liver is responsible for producing bile, which is used in the digestive process, as well as producing cholesterol and proteins. It also processes nutrients, medicines and alcohol, helping to cleanse the blood, and works to store glucose. Therefore, when its functioning is compromised, the patient may experience a series of imbalances in their metabolism and body. Cirrhosis is a chronic disease and has no cure. It is progressive and usually evolves gradually, and may not cause any symptoms at first.Cirrhosis is most commonly associated with excessive consumption of alcohol and other drugs, but it can also be the result of other diseases, such as autoimmune hepatitis B and C, which can be triggered by excessive use of certain medications.

The main causes of cirrhosis include

o excessive and continuous consumption of alcoholic beverages;

o excessive consumption of medication without following medical advice, known as drug hepatitis;

o diseases of viral origin, such as hepatitis B and hepatitis C;

o autoimmune diseases;

o Wilson's disease;

o Budd-Chiari syndrome;

o chronic cholestasis;

o biliary tract tumours.

What are the risk factors for developing cirrhosis?

There are some risk factors that can increase a patient's chances of developing cirrhosis. These include

o alcoholism, the continuous excessive consumption of alcoholic beverages;

o obesity;

o diabetes;

o hepatitis (types B, C and autoimmune);

o excessive and unregulated use of medication.

In general, any patient can have cirrhosis. However, the disease is more common in male patients. According to data from the Ministry of Health, cirrhosis was the 10th leading cause of death in Brazil in 2017. Liver cirrhosis is sometimes confused with primary biliary cirrhosis, but the two conditions are different. Primary biliary cirrhosis is the result of an inflammatory process that results in an accumulation of bile in the liver, with a different evolution to liver cirrhosis. Initially, cirrhosis has no symptoms. However, as the disease progresses and liver involvement increases, the main symptoms are: abdominal pain; nausea and vomiting; yellowing of the eyes and skin; swelling in the legs and abdomen, where some veins may be visible under the skin; ascites, which is the presence of water in the abdomen; dark urine; constipation; fatigue and tiredness. One of the most common complications of cirrhosis is hepatic encephalopathy, in which the brain can stop functioning properly, causing loss of consciousness and mental confusion due to problems with the liver. Cirrhosis also increases the patient's chance of liver cancer, infections in the body and haemorrhages and internal bleeding. There is no cure for cirrhosis and it is not possible to reverse the damage to the liver once it has set in.

Cirrhosis is treated in such a way as to prevent further damage to the liver, including by treating addiction, if this is the cause of the cirrhosis. Finally, in the most severe cases of cirrhosis, a liver transplant is required.

Before a liver transplant can be carried out, however, it is important to emphasise that the patient needs to undergo an assessment that will determine whether or not they are a viable candidate for a liver transplant. In this assessment, for example, the reasons that led the patient to cirrhosis are studied. In cases where the disease is caused by alcoholism or hepatitis B, the patient's current situation needs to be assessed to make sure there is no chance of cirrhosis compromising the new organ received in the liver transplant.

Hepatitis

Inflammation of the liver. It can be viral (hepatitis A, B, C, D and E), alcoholic or autoimmune (caused by the individual's own immune system). Hepatitis refers to any inflammation of the liver due to various causes, the most common of which are infections with type A, B and C viruses and the abuse of alcohol or other toxic substances (such as some medicines). While viruses attack the liver when they parasitise its cells in order to reproduce, cirrhosis in alcoholics is caused by frequent drinking - once in the body, alcohol is transformed into acids that are harmful to liver cells.

Types of liver failure:

Liver failure can be classified into different types according to the onset and progression of symptoms, the main ones being: Acute liver failure or acute liver failure: happens suddenly, 1 to 4 weeks after the liver injury, usually in healthy people with no previous liver disease. It is usually caused by the hepatitis virus or the incorrect use of certain medications, such as paracetamol; Chronic liver failure: symptoms can take months or even years to appear, and happen when the liver suffers constant aggression due to situations such as alcohol abuse, hepatitis or fatty liver;Acute chronic liver failure: caused by a decompensation of liver diseases, such as cirrhosis, due to factors such as alcohol consumption or infections, leading to the appearance of acute symptoms. Furthermore, liver failure can also be hyperacute, which appears in around 7 days, or subacute, which appears in 5 to 12 weeks, between the onset of symptoms and the development of hepatic encephalopathy. The type of liver failure is determined by the doctor by assessing the symptoms, as well as their onset, and tests that identify their cause.

Treatment:

Treatment for liver failure should be carried out under the guidance of a hepatologist or gastroenterologist and depends on the causes and stage of the disease. It should be done in hospital in an intensive care unit so that the person is constantly monitored to avoid complications.

Types:

Hepatitis A: is transmitted by contaminated water and food or from one person to another; the disease incubates for between 10 and 50 days and normally does not cause symptoms, but when present, the most common are fevers, yellowing of the skin and eyes, nausea and vomiting, malaise, abdominal discomfort, lack of appetite, Coca-Cola coloured urine and whitish stools. Detection is by blood test and there is no specific treatment, as the patient is expected to react to the disease on their own. Although there is a vaccine against the hepatitis A virus (HAV), the best way to prevent it is through basic sanitation, proper water treatment, well-cooked food and always washing your hands before meals. Hepatitis B and Hepatitis C: the type B (HBV) and type C (HCV) hepatitis viruses are transmitted mainly through blood. Injecting drug users and patients who have undergone contaminated and non-disposable surgical material are among the biggest victims, which is why care should be taken with blood transfusions, at the dentist's, during waxing or tattooing sessions. The hepatitis B virus can be passed on through sexual contact, reinforcing the need to use condoms. Often, the signs of hepatitis B and C don't appear and many of those infected only discover they have the disease after years and often by chance in tests for these viruses. When they do appear, the symptoms are very similar to those of hepatitis A, but unlike hepatitis A, B and C can develop into a chronic condition and then into cirrhosis or even liver cancer.

Treatment:

There is no treatment for the acute form. If necessary, only for symptoms such as nausea and vomiting. Rest is considered important due to the patient's condition. The use of a low-fat, high-carbohydrate diet is popular, but its main benefit is that it is better to digest for patients without an appetite. In practical terms, it should be recommended that the patient defines their diet according to their dietary preferences. The only restriction is on alcohol intake. This restriction should be maintained for at least six months and preferably a year.

Prevention:

The best strategy for preventing hepatitis A includes improving living conditions, improving basic sanitation and hygiene education measures. The specific vaccine against the A virus is indicated as recommended by the National Immunisation Programme (PNI). Prevention of hepatitis B includes effective control of blood banks through serological screening; vaccination against hepatitis B, available from SUS, as standardised by the National Immunisation Programme (PNI); the use of hepatitis B antivirus human immunoglobulin, also available from SUS, as standardised by the National Immunisation Programme (PNI); the use of personal protective equipment. by health professionals; not sharing nail clippers, razors, toothbrushes, equipment for drug use; the use of condoms in sexual relations. There is no vaccine to prevent hepatitis

C, but there are other forms of prevention, such as: screening in blood banks and semen donation centres to ensure the distribution of uninfected biological material; screening solid organ donors such as heart, liver, lung and kidney; screening cornea or skin donors; compliance with infection control practices in hospitals, laboratories, dental practices, haemodialysis services; treatment of infected individuals, when indicated; abstinence or reduced use of alcohol, no exposure to other substances that are toxic to the liver, such as certain medications.There are various types of hepatitis, including drug hepatitis. This is a disease characterised by inflammation of the liver cells caused by the use of medicines, as the name suggests, as well as illicit drugs, herbal medicines or even food supplements. For this reason, self-medication and improper use of substances can affect the organ.Medicinal hepatitis is an inflammation that affects the liver as a result of the use of drugs, medicines, food supplements, herbal medicines or plant products such as tea and herbs. The disease can be acute or chronic. In some cases, this type of hepatitis is caused by the excessive use of drugs that are toxic to the body (dose-dependent damage). In other situations, it can occur due to a person's hypersensitivity to a drug, which makes the organ more susceptible to this condition. Drug hepatitis is not a contagious disease.

Symptoms:

In most cases, drug hepatitis is asymptomatic and is detected in routine tests. When symptoms do appear, they can be: acute hepatitis with nausea; vomiting; tiredness; lack of appetite; jaundice (yellowing eyes and skin); dark, coffee-coloured urine. In rarer cases, the disease can develop into severe liver failure, i.e. the liver stops working properly and requires intensive care, so in some cases a liver transplant is urgently needed. In other cases, the disease can develop into chronic hepatitis or cirrhosis.

Medicinal hepatitis, as mentioned above, is an inflammation caused by the use of medicines or substances that are toxic to the body and affect liver cells. Antibiotics are the most common, as are anticonvulsants and anti-inflammatory drugs. In addition, teas, herbal remedies and stimulant tonics can also cause the condition. Although many people believe that natural products are not harmful to health, they can still be agents of contamination and contain toxic and infectious substances such as heavy metals.

The main causes of drug hepatitis are anti-inflammatories, antibiotics and anticonvulsants, herbal medicines and anabolic steroids, as mentioned above. It's worth emphasising that the same medication doesn't always affect everyone, as some people may be more sensitive than others to certain substances. That's why it's important to use medicines under medical supervision, to avoid overdosing or even misusing them, according to each organism.

The main risk factors for drug hepatitis are: the use of medication combined with alcohol; advanced age; previous liver disease; the use of plant extracts and high doses of medication To avoid drug hepatitis, only use medications and supplements with a doctor's prescription. In addition, avoid formulas with miraculous promises and the use of drugs in conjunction with the consumption of alcoholic beverages, and use medications for as short a time as possible and at the required dose.The most effective way to prevent drug hepatitis is to stop taking the suspected substance and not use it again. Around 90 per cent of cases improve spontaneously. Asymptomatic patients, on the other hand, need hydration and treatment to relieve symptoms such as itching, allergies, nausea and/or vomiting. And those who have impaired liver function should be referred to an intensive care unit with support and assessment for liver transplantation. It's important to inform your doctor about the use of medication in cases of suspected drug toxicity, even supplements, homemade herb a l products, teas and herbs. Then you need to follow the doctor's advice about using certain medicines or changing the type of medicine. The doctor may also order additional tests to diagnose toxic liver damage at an early stage.

Acute liver failure

Rapid decrease in liver function, which can be fatal. It is usually caused by poisoning, mainly through high doses of medication and contact with toxic substances. It can also appear as a complication of other liver diseases. Liver failure is the sudden or gradual loss of liver function, leading to symptoms such as nausea, vomiting, yellowing of the skin and eyes, swelling of the stomach, loss of appetite or excessive tiredness. Liver failure can be caused by liver diseases such as cirrhosis or hepatitis, or by frequent consumption of alcoholic beverages or the use of medicines such as paracetamol. Liver failure should be treated as soon as possible in hospital by a hepatologist, gastroenterologist or general practitioner, in order to avoid complications such as clotting problems, cerebral oedema or kidney failure. In some cases, medication or even liver transplantation may be indicated.

Symptoms:

The main symptoms of liver failure are: nausea; vomiting, which may contain blood; diarrhoea; loss of appetite; feeling full even after a light meal; excessive tiredness; pain in the upper right side of the abdomen; skin and eyes yellowing, known as jaundice; swelling in the belly; swelling in the legs; weight loss; sweet-smelling breath; dark urine; pale or whitish faeces; easy bruising or bleeding; itching in the body; mental confusion or disorientation; excessive drowsiness; general malaise.

The symptoms of liver failure can develop quickly, in days or weeks, which is called acute liver failure or acute kidney failure, or they can develop over time, over months or years, which is called chronic liver failure.

In the presence of symptoms of liver failure, it is important to consult a hepatologist or gastroenterologist as soon as possible or go to the nearest emergency room, as the disease can worsen rapidly and cause life-threatening haemorrhages or serious problems with the kidneys or brain.Liver failure is diagnosed by a gastroenterologist or hepatologist by assessing symptoms, health history and blood tests that measure blood clotting time, blood ammonia levels and liver enzymes such as ALT, AST, GGT, alkaline phosphatase and bilirubin. In addition, imaging tests of the abdomen, pelvis, brain and chest may be necessary, such as abdominal ultrasound with doppler, computerised tomography or magnetic resonance imaging, as well as a liver biopsy to check why this organ isn't working. See all the tests to assess liver function.In cases where there is no well-established cause, the doctor may also request a blood test for paracetamol levels, a toxicological test and a serological test for viruses.

Liver failure is caused by damage to the liver cells, interfering with the functioning of the liver and altering its functions. The main causes of liver failure are: viral hepatitis type A, B, C or E; frequent use of paracetamol or use in larger doses than recommended; excessive consumption of alcoholic beverages; cirrhosis of the liver; autoimmune hepatitis; use of medicinal plants such as kava-kava, ephedra, skullcap or pennyroyal; use of medicines such as antibiotics, anti-inflammatory or anticonvulsants; infection with the Epstein-Barr virus, cytomegalovirus, herpes simplex virus, parvovirus, adenovirus or varicella-zoster virus; Budd-Chiari syndrome, which can cause blockages in the veins of the liver; ischaemic hepatitis, which causes liver damage due to a decrease in the supply of oxygen to liver cells; Wilson's disease, in which copper accumulates in the liver; autoimmune diseases, such as autoimmune hepatitis; poisoning by the wild mushroom Amanita phalloides; liver cancer; metastasis in the liver from other types of cancer, such as breast cancer, lung cancer or lymphoma; generalised infection. In some cases, liver failure may have no apparent cause. In addition, acute liver failure can also occur in the third trimester of pregnancy when a woman has HELLP syndrome or acute fatty liver, which is why it is important to have medical monitoring during pregnancy.

Thus, the main treatments for liver failure are:

Use of medication

The drugs that the hepatologist or gastroenterologist can prescribe to treat liver failure depend on what caused the disease.
Some drugs that can be prescribed by a doctor for liver failure in hospital are:
o N-acetylcysteine, orally or intravenously, in case of paracetamol intoxication or other causes, except ischaemic hepatitis;
o Activated charcoal, suitable for use within 4 hours of accidental ingestion or large doses of paracetamol, or for Amanita phalloides poisoning;
o Antivirals, such as acyclovir, gancivlovir or lamivudine, to treat acute hepatitis B, varicella-zoster, herpes simplex or cytomegalovirus;
o Steroids, such as injectable prednisolone, in the case of autoimmune hepatitis;
o Penicillamine, for the treatment of Wilson's disease;
o Penicillin G into the vein in case of mushroom poisoning;
o Antibiotics, in case of generalised infection or sepsis;
o Vasopressors, such as dopamine or norepinephrine in the vein, in cases of very low blood pressure.

The doctor may also prescribe other remedies depending on the illness and symptoms.

Monitoring:

During hospitalisation, the person is constantly monitored in order to avoid complications such as hepatic encephalopathy, cerebral oedema, bleeding, infections or kidney failure.

This way, if the person shows changes in the monitoring, they can be indicated:

o Use of a catheter in the brain to monitor intracranial pressure, elevation of the headboard to 45°, or use of mannitol in the vein if there are changes in intracranial pressure;

o Endotracheal intubation in cases of hepatic encephalopathy greater than grade 2, intestinal lavage or use of laxatives;

o Transfusions of platelets or fresh plasma, or use of vitamin K in the vein, in cases of bleeding or haemorrhage;

o Dialysis or haemodialysis in case of kidney failure.

In addition, if the doctor detects a drop in blood glucose, it may be recommended to administer glucose serum into the vein.

Make changes to your diet:

The diet for liver failure should be carried out under the supervision of a hepatologist and a clinical nutritionist, as the guidelines depend on the person's state of health and the stage of the disease. In general, you should control the amount of fluids you drink, restrict your salt intake to less than 2g a day to avoid swelling or fluid accumulation in the abdomen, and not drink alcoholic beverages as they can worsen symptoms and aggravate the disease.

Liver transplant:

Liver transplantation is a surgery that removes the liver that no longer functions properly and replaces it with a healthy liver from a deceased donor or a part of a healthy liver from a living donor. This treatment, when carried out in time, can restore liver function. However, it is not indicated in all cases, such as liver failure caused by hepatitis, as the virus can take hold in the transplanted liver. Find out how liver transplants are carried out.

The main complications of liver failure are: hepatic encephalopathy; cerebral oedema; gastrointestinal haemorrhage; bacterial or fungal infection; pulmonary oedema; renal failure. These complications can arise soon after the first symptoms of the disease or when the disease is at a more advanced stage, and must be treated immediately, because if they are not reversed or controlled in time, they can be life-threatening.

Liver cancer

It can originate in the liver or be the result of a metastasis of a cancer that began in another organ. Its main risk factors are chronic hepatitis B or C and Malignant liver tumours can be divided into two types: primary cancer (which originates in the organ itself) and secondary or metastatic cancer (which originates in another organ and also affects the liver). Among tumours originating in the liver, the most common is hepatocarcinoma or hepatocellular carcinoma. Aggressive, it occurs in more than 80 per cent of cases. Other types of primary liver cancer are cholangiocarcinoma (originating in the liver's bile ducts), angiosarcoma (a rare cancer that originates in the organ's blood vessels) and hepatoblastoma, a rare malignant tumour that affects newborns and children in the first few years of life.

Symptoms:

Abdominal pain, abdominal mass, distension, unexplained weight loss, loss of appetite, malaise, jaundice (yellowish tinge to the skin and eyes) and ascites (accumulation of fluid in the abdomen).

Diagnosis:

Due to the short evolution time of hepatocarcinoma, the tumour is usually advanced when the diagnosis is made. The average doubling time of the mass is four months. Some tests will help the doctor confirm the diagnosis: computed tomography: a test that uses X-rays and computer technology to produce images as if it were a "slice" of the body and serves to discover and locate tumours, magnetic resonance imaging (MRI): does not differ greatly from computed tomography in terms of its ability to identify primary or metastatic liver tumours. This test can define the extent of the tumour a little better in patients with liver cirrhosis.

Laparoscopy also allows direct visualisation of the organ and biopsy (removal of a small amount of tissue for laboratory analysis to determine whether the tumour is malignant or not). It is most effective when combined with laparoscopic ultrasound.

Treatment:

Surgical removal (resection) of the tumour is the most indicated treatment when the tumour is restricted to a part of the liver (primary tumour) and also in metastatic liver tumours where the primary lesion has been resected or is amenable to curative resection.

Prevention:

Cirrhosis of the liver is the cause of half of all cases of hepatocarcinoma. Cirrhosis, in turn, is associated with alcoholism or chronic hepatitis, the most common cause of which is infection with the hepatitis B or C viruses. In order not to develop cirrhosis of the liver, you need to control the amount of alcohol you drink, never exceeding two doses a day. Transmission of the hepatitis B virus can be prevented by vaccination.

Eating a diet high in fibre (whole grains, cereals, vegetables and fruit) and low in saturated fats prevents various types of cancer, such as bowel, rectal, breast and lung cancer, which are known to metastasise to the liver. However, attention must be paid to the origin of grains and cereals, as when stored in inappropriate and damp places they can be contaminated by the fungus Aspergillus flavus, which produces the carcinogenic substance aflatoxin, a risk factor for hepatocarcinoma.

Cholangiocarcinoma

It is related to inflammation of the bile ducts, mainly due to infestation by a parasite of the digestive tract (clonorchis sinensis), which is very common in Asian and African countries.

Angiocarcinoma

Associated with the carcinogenic potential of chemical substances such as vinyl chloride, used in the manufacture of some types of plastic, inorganic arsenicals and Thorotrast (thorium dioxide solution).

Parasitosis

Various parasites can migrate to the liver and cause lesions or blockages, such as the worms that cause malaria and schistosomiasis, among others.

Prevention:

A few simple actions can help prevent most of the problems that affect the liver: always use condoms correctly, sanitise and cook food properly, keep your vaccinations up to date, protect yourself with gloves and other safety materials when you need to handle chemicals, maintain healthy lifestyle habits: exercise, eat a balanced diet and consume alcohol in moderation.

Treatment:

Liver disease can be treated with medication, but milder cases are only treated with changes to your diet and routine. In specific cases, surgery may be necessary. It all depends on the speed and accuracy of the diagnosis. When diagnosed early, most liver diseases can be cured before complications arise. Each diagnosis will require a different treatment, so it's important to look for a good clinic with good professionals. A good diagnosis will include imaging tests such as ultrasounds and MRI scans, laboratory tests and a biopsy when necessary.

CHAPTER 3

MARKERS OF LIVER DAMAGE

ANA PATRICIA DE OLIVEIRA JANAINA MAIA LIMA ROSAL
BRUNA DA SILVA SOUZA

Biochemical Liver Markers

The use of serum biochemical tests plays an important role in the diagnosis and treatment of liver diseases. However, an isolated test provides limited information, which must be evaluated in the context of the patient's history and clinical condition. Liver biochemical tests consist of hepatocellular injury markers (aminotransferases and alkaline phosphatase), liver metabolism tests (bilirubin) and liver synthetic function tests (serum albumin and prothrombin time - PT). The liver contains a high concentration of enzymes, some of which are present in the serum in very low concentrations. Injury to the hepatocyte membrane leads to extravasation of these enzymes into the serum, which results in an increase in serum concentration within a few hours of liver damage.Serum enzyme tests can be categorised into two groups: enzymes whose elevation reflects generalised hepatocyte damage (aminotransferases) and enzymes whose elevation mainly reflects cholestasis (alkaline phosphatase, gamma-glutamyltransferase or gamma-glutamyltranspeptidase -GGT). Aminotransferases (formerly called transaminases) are sensitive indicators of hepatocyte damage. They consist of aspartate aminotransferase (AST) and alanine aminotransferase (ALT). AST is found in decreasing order of concentration in the liver, heart muscle, skeletal muscle, kidneys, brain, pancreas, lungs, leucocytes and erythrocytes. ALT, on the other hand, is present in higher concentrations in the liver, making it a more specific marker for liver damage.

Alkaline phosphatase represents a group of enzymes present in practically all tissues. It has four subtypes according to its localisation (intestinal, placental, liver, bone and kidney). As alkaline phosphatase is present in different tissues, isolated elevations do not always mean liver disease.

Diseases of the bone, small intestine and even pregnancy can cause an isolated increase. The main value of serum alkaline phosphatase in diagnosing liver disease is in recognising cholestatic disease. In patients with cholestasis, alkaline phosphatase is typically elevated by at least four times the upper limit of normal. GGT is an enzyme found in hepatocytes and biliary epithelial cells, as well as in the kidneys, prostate, pancreas, spleen, heart and brain. It is used to find out if there is any organic damage, drug and/or medication intoxication, alcohol abuse or pancreatic disease.Lactate dehydrogenase (LDH) is a cytoplasmic enzyme present in tissues throughout the body. This test is not as sensitive as serum aminotransferases in liver disease and has low diagnostic specificity. It is more useful as a marker of haemolysis. It is elevated in cases of ischaemic hepatitis and, when accompanied by elevated alkaline FA-phosphatase, suggests malignant infiltration of the liver. The rupture of red blood cells releases haemoglobin, which is taken up by the reticulo-endothelial system of the liver, spleen and bone marrow and transformed by hemeoxygenase into biliverdin. Biliverdin reductase converts biliverdin into free bilirubin.

This form of bilirubin is called unconjugated or indirect (IB) and is fat-soluble.

BI binds to albumin, the form in which it is transported in the plasma, taken up by the hepatocyte and transported to the endoplasmic reticulum, where it is converted by the action of the enzyme uridine diphosphataseglycuronosyl-transferase into conjugated or direct bilirubin (BD). BD is transported through the canalicular membrane into the bile, and is one of the stages that are more susceptible to impairment in the event of liver damage. Once excreted from the hepatocyte into the bile duct, BD is transported via the bile ducts to the duodenum. Increases in BI may be due to increased production, decreased uptake and/or conjugation by the hepatocyte, while increases in BD are generally due to hepatocellular or biliary dysfunction. In the neonatal period, there may be a physiological increase in BI. However, it is recommended to measure total bilirubin and fractions in all children who remain jaundiced after the second week of life.

Unlike indirect hyperbilirubinaemia, which can be physiological, elevated BD is always correlated with pathological conditions and reflects a decrease in bile secretion due to hepatocellular or biliary disease, i.e. cholestasis. Any newborn or infant with a BD > 1.0 mg/dl deserves diagnostic investigation. This is an urgent condition and must be identified early by the paediatrician. The normal concentration of total serum bilirubin is less than 1 mg/dl. The direct fraction corresponds to up to 30 per cent of the total, or 0.3 mg/dl. Albumin is the most abundant plasma protein and is responsible for 80 per cent of plasma osmotic pressure. Due to its long half-life of around 21 days, its levels may not be affected in acute liver diseases, such as viral hepatitis or liver failure of any aetiology.In cirrhosis or chronic liver disease, low serum albumin can be a sign of advanced liver disease. However, low serum albumin is not specific to liver disease and can occur in other conditions, such as malnutrition, infections, nephrotic syndrome or protein-losing enteropathy. Normal serum albumin concentrations are between 3.5 g/dl and 5.0 g/dl. The prothrombin time (PT) and INR (international normalised ratio) measure the activity of coagulation factors I, II, V, VII and X, which are all synthesised in the liver and dependent on vitamin K for synthesis. Coagulation factors have a much shorter half-life than albumin. For this reason, PT/NI is the best measure of the liver's synthetic function in acute conditions.PT prolongation of more than 5 seconds above the control value (INR > 1.5) is a sign of poor liver disease prognosis and an important factor in prioritising liver transplantation. It is not a sensitive indicator in chronic liver disease, as even in cases of severe cirrhosis, levels can be normal or slightly increased. Vitamin K deficiency also causes prolonged PT and can be due to malnutrition, malabsorption and severe cholestasis with an inability to absorb fat-soluble vitamins. The administration of vitamin K can help distinguish vitamin K deficiency from hepatocyte dysfunction, as replacement results in the correction of PT in the case of vitamin K deficiency, but not in liver dysfunction.

CHAPTER 4

LIVER CAUSED BY MEDICATION

ANA PATRICIA DE OLIVEIRA JANAINA MAIA LIMA ROSAL

BRUNA DA SILVA SOUZA

Hepatotoxicity or drug-induced liver damage can be defined as damage to the liver caused by medications or toxins that can lead to abnormalities in liver laboratory tests up to fulminant liver failure with acute liver necrosis and the need for liver transplantation.

Drug-induced liver damage accounts for around 30 per cent of acute hepatitis worldwide and 10 per cent of adverse drug reactions, and is the biggest reason for medication withdrawals. It is difficult to assess the true frequency and incidence of drug-induced liver damage due to the difficulty in establishing the cause and the retrospective nature of the studies. Paracetamol intoxication is relatively common, due to its ready availability, and because it is present in combination products, such as the antipyretics prescribed in the United States and countries around the world.

They are classified into

Mechanism of toxicity: predictable or idiosyncratic. Most medications cause liver damage by an idiosyncratic mechanism, in other words, it doesn't depend on the dose used, except for paracetamol and methotrexate, which don't usually cause liver damage, except at doses higher than those prescribed in usual doses. Paracetamol hepatoxicity, for example, only causes liver damage in high doses, after ingestion of 7.5 to 10g over an 8-hour period. Clinical presentation: hepatocellular damage (damage to the hepatocytes), cholestatic damage (the name given to the reduction in the flow of bile, either due to impaired secretion in the hepatocytes or due to a reduction or interruption in this flow) and mixed damage. The liver is the main organ responsible for metabolising medicines and toxins. Ingested compounds are absorbed from the gastrointestinal tract and transported to the liver via the portal circulation. Most human toxins are lipophilic. Therefore, in order to be excreted through the urine or bile, an enzymatic modification is required within the hepatocytes to make it water-soluble. Around 50 per cent of cases of hepatotoxicity are of the hepatocellular lesion type, such as that which occurs in the case of paracetamol intoxication, acute iron toxicity or exposure to halogenated hydrocarbons (e.g. carbon tetrachloride and halothane).

Chronic cholestasis is more common with drugs such as statins (cholesterol-lowering medication), azathioprine, bupropion, carbamazepine, antidepressants such as mirtazapine and tricyclics. Hepatic steatosis refers to the abnormal presence of lipids inside hepatocytes. Chronic use of some drugs can cause liver cirrhosis, such as alphamethyldopa (antihypertensive) and methotrexate (used in rheumatological diseases). Methotrexate-induced cirrhosis is dose-dependent and does not occur with cumulative doses of less than 1 to 2 grams. Caution should be exercised in the indiscriminate use of herbal medicines such as tea, herbs and nutritional supplements. These medicines can also cause hepatotoxicity, such as thermogenic and Herbalife products used for weight loss. Nowadays, the practice of treating illnesses with herbs and teas is attracting an increasingly large market. In the United States alone, the natural medicines market mobilises more than 180 billion dollars, with sales of more than 6 billion dollars a year in nutritional supplements. Of this amount, at least 1 billion sales a year revolve around teas and herbs alone.

The main risk factors are older age (increases the risk of developing cholestatic lesions), female gender (as they usually have a smaller body surface area, they are at greater risk of drug-induced hepatotoxicity, especially of the autoimmune type), alcohol use (alcohol can increase toxicity in patients with repeated supratherapeutic doses of acetaminophen, methotrexate and tuberculostatic drugs), and an increase in previous TGP (liver enzyme) levels, comorbidities such as diabetes, hepatitis B and C, psoriasis, obesity and pregnant women. African Americans have an increased risk of hepatotoxicity with anticonvulsants. Younger patients are at greater risk of hepatotoxicity of valproic acid and salicylates, as well as drug-related hepatocellular damage in general.Symptoms can be non-specific, such as asthenia, anorexia, nausea, abdominal pain, fever, jaundice, choluria and pruritus, as well as a slight increase in transaminases (liver enzymes) without evidence of liver failure, which are commonly observed in emergency assessments. In severe cases, the patient may progress to severe acute liver failure (SAHF), also known as fulminant hepatitis, which is defined as the onset of hepatic encephalopathy within two weeks of the onset of symptoms of liver toxicity (jaundice), in which case liver transplantation is the only treatment.The initial approach to clinical assessment involves a thorough history and physical examination. A history of medication intake, as well as recently consumed food, herbal and supplement products should be obtained. Careful assessment should include blood tests to assess liver function such as TGO/TGP/FA/GGT and coagulation such as full blood count with platelets and INR. Other tests are requested depending on the clinical context of the presentation and situations such as in cases of paracetamol intoxication, which have specific indications for complementary tests. The main management measure for these patients is the withdrawal of the drug that caused the initial process and supportive treatment for complications of liver disease. There are rare situations in which specific measures need to be adopted, such as paracetamol intoxication. Sometimes the process of improvement is slow, and in some cases there may be a worsening of liver function even after drug withdrawal, requiring liver transplantation.

CHAPTER 5

RECOMMENDED TREATMENT FOR LIVER DAMAGE

ANA PATRICIA DE OLIVEIRA JANAINA MAIA LIMA ROSAL

BRUNA DA SILVA SOUZA

Liver diseases can have a complex effect on the clearance, biotransformation and pharmacokinetics of drugs. Pathogenic factors include changes in intestinal absorption, plasma protein binding, hepatic extraction rate, hepatic blood flow and systemic port shunts, biliary excretion, enterohepatic circulation and renal clearance.By increasing the bioavailability levels of a drug, these alterations can lead it to cause possible toxic effects even at normal doses. However, levels and effects for a particular drug are unpredictable and do not necessarily correlate with the type of liver injury or disease, its severity, or even the results of liver tests. Therefore, no general rule is available for adjusting dosage in patients with liver disease. Clinical effects can vary independently of the bioavailability of the drug, especially in chronic hepatopathies; e.g. in chronic hepatopathies, cerebral sensitivity to opioids and sedatives is generally better. Thus, apparently small doses of these drugs administered to patients with cirrhosis can precipitate encephalopathy. The mechanism explaining this effect probably involves alterations in brain drug receptors. Adverse reactions to drugs are no more likely to occur in patients with liver disease, but these patients may tolerate any adverse hepatic effects of drugs less well. The body has to process (chemically alter or metabolise) medicines so that it can use and eliminate them. Much of this processing takes place in the liver and is carried out by liver enzymes. Medicines and the liver are therefore interconnected in many ways:

o Liver disorders can alter the way a drug is metabolised;

o Some medicines can damage the liver;

o Many factors (such as the food eaten, a person's genetics and the use of other drugs) can affect how the liver metabolises drugs (see Factors that affect drug response).

Medicines can affect how quickly other medicines are metabolised in the liver. If a medicine is metabolised more quickly, it can be broken down and eliminated before it performs its function. In the case of drugs with a slower metabolism, side effects are more likely.

Liver disorders often alter the effect of medicines in the body - for example, by altering..:

o The amount of medicine absorbed from the intestine;

o How quickly and efficiently a drug is metabolised by the liver - for example, changing the drug into an active or inactive form (a form that has no effect on the body);

o The amount of medicine transported throughout the body;

o How quickly the drug is eliminated from the body;

o The body's sensitivity to the effects of medicines.

The way in which liver disorders affect a medicine depends on the type of medicine. Liver disorders can increase the effects of some medicines and decrease the effects of others. The effect of the medicine is increased if the liver is less able to inactivate a medicine.

The effect of the medicine is decreased if the liver is less able to change it into the active form or if the liver makes the body less able to absorb the medicine or transport it through the body. Liver disorders can increase the effects of some medicines and decrease the effects of others. A chronic liver disorder can make people more sensitive to the effects of certain medicines, even when the disorder does not increase the amount of medicine in the body.

For example, if people with certain liver disorders take even small doses of opioid painkillers (such as morphine) or sedatives (such as lorazepam), their mental functioning can deteriorate, and they can become confused, disorientated and less alert. Mental functioning deteriorates probably because the liver disorder makes the brain more sensitive to the effects of these drugs.

Because liver disorders are complicated, doctors often can't predict how they will affect a particular drug. It can therefore be difficult to adjust drug doses in people with liver disorders. Many medicines can affect the functioning of the liver or can damage it, or both.

Some drugs, such as statins (used to treat high cholesterol), can increase liver enzyme levels and cause liver damage (usually minor), but without symptoms. However, doctors can continue to prescribe statins for people with chronic liver disease (e.g. non-alcoholic fatty liver disease [NAFLD], non-alcoholic steatohepatitis [NASH] and cirrhosis caused by NASH), because statins do not pose a greater risk for these people compared to those without liver disease and there are benefits to using statins to treat high cholesterol in people with NAFLD and NASH. However, statins are not prescribed, or are prescribed in lower doses, for many people with decompensated cirrhosis (an advanced stage of cirrhosis in which the liver can no longer function properly).A very small number of drugs damage the liver enough to cause symptoms such as yellowing skin (jaundice), abdominal pain, itching and a tendency to bruise and bleed. Doctors use the term drug-induced liver injury (DILI) to refer to any liver damage caused by medication, regardless of whether or not it causes symptoms. This term also includes damage caused by illicit drugs, medicinal herbs, plants and nutritional supplements. In the case of some drugs, liver damage is predictable. It occurs soon after the drug is ingested and is dose-related. In the United States, this damage (often caused by paracetamol intoxication) is one of the most common causes of the sudden onset of jaundice, liver failure or both. For other drugs, the damage is unpredictable. It is detected some time after the drug is ingested and is not dose-related. Rarely, these lesions result in a serious liver disorder.

Some medicinal herbs (parts of the plant used for health benefits) contain substances that can damage the liver. The liver is a prime target for damage because it processes everything that is ingested through the mouth.

Hundreds of herbs contain pyrrolizidine alkaloids, which can damage the liver. These herbs include borage, comfrey and certain Chinese herbs, such as zi cao (Radix arnabiae), kuan dong hua (tussilago), qian li guang (root of life) and pei lan (Eupatorium). Some herbs used to make teas contain pyrrolizidine alkaloids. Sometimes milk, honey and cereals are contaminated with pyrrolizidine alkaloids, which can then be ingested unknowingly. They can damage the liver gradually if small amounts are consumed over a prolonged period of time. Damage can occur more quickly if a large amount is consumed. The hepatic veins can become obstructed, blocking blood flow out of the liver.

Affected people experience abdominal pain and may vomit. Fluid accumulates in the abdomen and legs. Eventually, scar tissue in the liver (cirrhosis), liver failure and even death can occur.

Liver damage can also be caused by herbs such as Atractylis gummifera, Camellia sinensis (used to make black tea and green tea), celandine (from the poppy family), chaparral, Garcinia cambogia (a supplement used to support weight loss), green tea extract (used for weight loss and disease prevention), germander, jin bu huan, kava, ma huang (Ephedra), bird's-foot trefoil, pennyroyal oil (used to make teas) and syo-saiko-to (a mixture of herbs).

In general, liver doctors (hepatologists) recommend avoiding all herbal supplements due to the lack of safety tests by the US Food and Drug Administration (FDA) and the fact that many of these substances can cause liver damage and even liver failure, even in people without pre-existing liver disease.

It is generally believed that the risk of liver damage from medication is increased by the following: age (18 or over), obesity, pregnancy, alcohol consumption or a genetic makeup that makes people more susceptible to the effects of a medication.Drinking alcohol increases the risk of liver damage because alcohol damages the liver and therefore alters the way medicines are metabolised. In addition, alcohol reduces the body's supply of an antioxidant that helps protect the liver. Doctors categorise drug-induced liver damage in various ways, for example, how the drug damages the liver, how the hepatocytes are affected and what liver enzyme abnormalities are detected by blood tests. For example, drugs can damage the liver by directly damaging the hepatocytes (hepatocellular), by blocking the flow of bile out of the liver (cholestatic) or both.

Medicines that can damage the liver:The symptoms of liver disease range from general (such as fatigue, a general feeling of malaise, nausea, itching and loss of appetite) to more serious symptoms (such as jaundice, an enlarged liver, pain in the upper right part of the abdomen, confusion, disorientation and reduced attention).Diagnosis of drug-related liver damage is usually based on medical assessment and tests, such as blood tests or imaging tests. After discontinuing If the drug is suspected of causing the injury, doctors repeat the liver function tests. A significant reduction in the level of liver enzymes further supports the diagnosis of drug-induced liver damage. If drug-induced liver damage is identified quickly, people have a better prognosis.Doctors ask which medications are being taken to determine whether any of them could be the cause of the liver damage. Doctors also order blood tests to measure the levels of specific liver enzymes and to assess how the liver is functioning and whether it is damaged (liver function tests).Drug-induced liver injury (DILI) is more likely when the results of liver function tests are characteristic of liver injury, usually caused by a drug that the person is taking. Medicines sometimes cause damage after they have been stopped, even when the dose was not high; and sometimes it can take several months for an ILD to improve. Therefore, determining that a drug is the cause can be difficult or impossible. As no test can confirm the diagnosis, doctors also check for other causes of liver damage. Blood tests are carried out to check for hepatitis, autoimmune diseases and other causes. Pressing on the upper abdomen to determine the size of the liver and diagnostic imaging tests such as ultrasound or computerised tomography (CT) can also help the doctor identify other causes of liver damage. The main treatment for drug-related liver damage is: stopping the drug, administration of the antidote if available, sometimes corticosteroids and sometimes liver transplantation, depending on its severity. Generally, discontinuing the drug results in recovery. Medicines that relieve symptoms, such as itching, can be used.Few medicines have antidotes. For example, N-acetylcysteine can be used if a person has overdosed on paracetamol. In some cases, the use of corticosteroids may be appropriate. If the damage is severe, the patient can be referred to a specialist. Liver transplantation may be necessary. When some drugs that can damage the liver (such as statins) are used, doctors regularly carry out blood tests to monitor liver enzyme levels. This monitoring can detect problems at an early stage and help prevent liver damage. For most drugs, monitoring of liver enzyme levels is not carried out.

REFERENCES

BERTONI G E., TREVISI X. H., BIONAZ M. Effects of Inflammatory Conditions on Liver Activity in Puerperium Period and Consequences for Performance in Dairy Cows.
J. Dairy Sci. 91:3300-3310, 2008.

DYCE K. M., SACK M. O., WENSING C.J. G. Tratado de anatomia veterinária, 3 ed., Elsevier, Rio de Janeiro, ch. 28, p. 663-664, 2004.

GONZALEZ F.H.D, SILVA S.C. Introdução à bioquímica clínica veterinária. 2ª ed. Porto Alegre:Editora da Universidade Federal do Rio Grande do Sul. c. 8, p. 318-337, 2006.

GUYTON Arthur C., Tratado de Fisiologia Médica, M, 9 ed., Guanabara Koogan, Rio de Janeiro, c. 70, p. 672, 1997.

MATTOS A. A. Tratado de hepatologia, 1 ed. Rubio, Rio de Janeiro, p. 960, 2010.

THRALL M.A. et. al. Hematology and veterinary clinical biochemistry, 2 ed., Guanabara Koogan, Rio de Janeiro, p. 349 to 360, 2015.

TREVISI, E., CALAMARI, L., BERTONI, G. Definition of the liver activity index in dairy cows and its relationship with reproductive performance. X Int. Symp . Vet. Lab. Diagnost, Salsomaggiore Parma, Italy; p. 118, 2001.

GREEM RM, FLAMM S. AGA Technical Review on the Evaluation of Liver Chemistry Tests. Gastroenterology 2002; 123:1367-84.

NEWSOME PN, CRAMB R, DAVISON MS, DILLON FJ, FOULERTON M,

GODFREY ME et al. Guidelines on the management of abnormal liver blood tests. Gut 2018; 67(1):6-19.

KWO PY, COHEN SM, LIM JK. ACG Clinical Guideline: Evaluation of Abnormal Liver Chemistries. Am J Gastroenterol 2017; 112:18.
BUSSLER S, VOGEL M, PIETZNER D et al. New paediatric percentiles of liver enzyme serum levels (alanine aminotransferase, aspartate aminotransferase, y- glutamyltransferase): Effects of age, sex, body mass index, and pubertal stage. Hepatology 2018; 68:1319-30.
ESTEY MP, COHEN AH, COLANTONIO DA, CHAN MK, MARVASTI TB, RANDELL E et al. CLSI-based transference of the CALIPER database of paediatric reference intervals from Abbott to Beckman, Ortho, Roche and Siemens Clinical Chemistry Assays: Direct validation using reference samples from the CALIPER cohort. Clin Biochem 2013; 46:1197-219.
LEE NG V. Laboratory assessment of Liver Function and Injury in Children. In: Suchy FJ, Sokol RJ, Balistreri WF, Bezerra JA, Mack CL, Shneider BL (eds). Liver Disease in Children. 5. ed. Cambridge: Cambridge University Press, 2021. p.94-105

CONTENTS

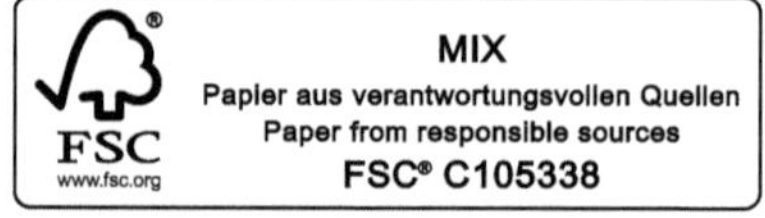